Wilson Disease

Coping with a Rare Genetic Disorder and Preventing Organ Damage

Key Information on Copper Accumulation, Liver Health, Symptoms, Treatment options, and Dietary Adjustments for Lifelong Management and Symptom Control

Graham Julian Oliver

Disclaimer

The information provided in this book, "Wilson Disease - Coping with a Rare Genetic Disorder and Preventing Organ Damage," is intended for general informational purposes only and is not a substitute for professional medical advice, diagnosis, or treatment. Always seek the advice of your physician or other qualified health provider with any questions you may have regarding a medical condition or treatment.

The author and publisher of this book do not endorse or recommend any specific individual, product, website, organization, or other names mentioned within. Any references to specific products, services, or organizations are for informational purposes only and do not constitute an endorsement. Reliance on any information provided in this book is solely at your own risk.

This book may contain descriptions of treatments, dietary adjustments, and health management strategies related to Wilson Disease and its symptoms. However, individual experiences with Wilson Disease can vary greatly. The author does not guarantee any specific outcomes, and the information in this book should not be considered as a substitute for personalized medical advice or treatment plans tailored to individual circumstances.

The author and publisher are not responsible for any claims, losses, or damages resulting from the use of or reliance on any information contained in this book.

About This Book

The book titled *Wilson Disease: Coping with a Rare Genetic Disorder and Preventing Organ Damage* serves as a crucial resource for individuals and families affected by Wilson Disease, offering comprehensive insights into a condition that disrupts copper metabolism in the body. With its focus on key information regarding copper accumulation, liver health, symptoms, treatment options, and dietary adjustments, this guide is indispensable for lifelong management and symptom control. It lays a solid foundation for understanding the implications of Wilson Disease, emphasizing the importance of proactive engagement in one's health journey.

Understanding Wilson Disease is pivotal for effective management, and the book provides a clear definition of this genetic disorder. By explaining how mutations in the ATP7B gene lead to the accumulation of copper, it illuminates the biological mechanisms that underlie the condition. The text details the critical consequences of this accumulation, such as liver damage and neurological issues, underscoring the urgency of early detection and intervention. This resource highlights the profound impact of lifestyle modifications and dietary adjustments, essential components for managing symptoms and mitigating complications effectively.

Early diagnosis is paramount in preventing severe health complications, a theme that resonates throughout the text. The book discusses the symptoms of Wilson Disease, which range from fatigue and jaundice to neurological disturbances like tremors and mood swings. It further emphasizes the importance of routine screenings and genetic testing, especially for individuals with a family history of the disorder. By promoting a multidisciplinary approach to diagnosis, the book encourages collaboration among healthcare providers to ensure timely and accurate identification of the disease.

The section on copper accumulation and liver health explores the vital role of the liver in regulating copper levels. It explains how excess copper can lead to liver dysfunction, the significance of liver enzyme tests, and the importance of imaging studies for monitoring liver health. Moreover, the potential complications of untreated Wilson Disease, including cirrhosis and the need for liver transplantation, are addressed, reinforcing the importance of regular check-ups and lifestyle modifications to maintain liver integrity.

Treatment options presented in the book, such as chelating therapy and zinc therapy, offer hope and direction for those managing Wilson Disease. The author provides detailed information on common chelating agents, their purpose, and possible side effects, ensuring that patients and their families understand the intricacies of their treatment plans. This resource also highlights the importance of adherence to prescribed therapies and the role of supportive care in symptom management, equipping readers with the knowledge needed to navigate their healthcare journeys confidently.

Dietary adjustments are crucial in managing Wilson Disease, and the book thoroughly discusses the dietary changes necessary for effective symptom control.

Readers will find lists of high-copper foods to avoid and recommendations for a low-copper diet. The importance of hydration and balanced nutrition is emphasized, along with tips for meal planning and understanding food labels. By involving a dietitian and fostering family support, individuals can make informed dietary choices that contribute to their overall health and well-being.

Lifestyle changes are also essential for managing Wilson Disease. The text encourages readers to adopt regular medical check-ups, stress management techniques, and exercise routines that promote overall health. It highlights the importance of social support, hydration, and maintaining a health journal, which can be instrumental in managing the daily challenges posed by the disorder. Engaging in hobbies and activities that promote mental health is strongly encouraged, providing readers with strategies to enrich their lives despite the diagnosis.

The book also delves into coping mechanisms, recognizing the emotional toll that chronic illness can take on individuals and their families. By promoting mental health awareness, it offers strategies for managing anxiety and depression, including the importance of therapy and support groups. The discussion surrounding communication with loved ones and educating them about Wilson Disease is vital for fostering understanding and empathy in relationships. Techniques for self-advocacy in healthcare and resources for mental health support empower readers to navigate their health challenges effectively.

Managing complications associated with Wilson Disease is another key focus of the book. It outlines potential complications, such as neurological damage, and emphasizes the importance of regular evaluations by specialists. Readers are equipped with strategies to recognize warning signs and navigate healthcare systems, ensuring they remain informed and proactive in managing their health. The inclusion of emergency protocols and patient advocacy resources further enhances the book's practicality.

Finally, the narrative of living with Wilson Disease is one of resilience and hope. The text encourages acceptance and adaptation, celebrating small victories along the health journey. It stresses the importance of community involvement and sharing experiences to foster a sense of belonging and support. Through patient stories of hope and perseverance, readers are inspired to embrace their lives fully while remaining committed to lifelong learning about Wilson Disease.

In summary, this book is an essential guide for anyone affected by Wilson Disease. By providing a wealth of information on the intricacies of copper metabolism, the significance of early diagnosis, treatment options, dietary adjustments, and coping mechanisms, it empowers readers to take charge of their health and well-being. Through knowledge and support, individuals with Wilson Disease can navigate their journey with confidence and resilience.

Table of Contents

Introduction

Definition of Wilson Disease as a Genetic Disorder Affecting Copper Metabolism

Wilson Disease is a rare genetic disorder characterized by the body's inability to properly metabolize copper. This condition is inherited in an autosomal recessive manner, meaning a person must inherit two copies of the defective gene—one from each parent—for the disorder to manifest. The ATP7B gene, responsible for copper transport and regulation, is typically mutated in individuals with Wilson Disease. As a result, copper accumulates in the liver, brain, and other organs, leading to a variety of health problems.

To understand Wilson Disease, it is important to recognize that the body requires a certain amount of copper for essential functions, but excess copper is toxic. Regular screening for symptoms, especially in individuals with a family history of the disease, can facilitate early diagnosis and treatment. Genetic testing can confirm the diagnosis, making it vital for affected individuals and their families to undergo testing and counseling for informed decision-making about health and lifestyle choices.

How Copper Accumulation Can Lead to Liver Damage and Neurological Issues

Copper accumulation in the body primarily affects the liver, where it can cause liver damage, cirrhosis, and ultimately liver failure if left untreated. Initially, the liver attempts to store excess copper, but when it becomes overwhelmed, copper leaks into the bloodstream, affecting other organs such as the brain. This leakage can lead to severe neurological symptoms, including tremors, speech difficulties, and personality changes, which may become progressively worse over time.

To prevent liver damage and manage neurological issues, early intervention is crucial. Regular medical check-ups, liver function tests, and monitoring of copper levels can help track the disease's progression. Patients often benefit from a multi-disciplinary care approach involving hepatologists, neurologists, and dietitians to address the complex health challenges associated with Wilson Disease. Early treatment strategies, including medication to reduce copper levels, can significantly improve outcomes and quality of life.

The Importance of Early Detection and Management

Early diagnosis of Wilson Disease is crucial for effective management and prevention of severe health complications. Identifying the disease in its initial stages allows for timely interventions, which can significantly reduce the risk of organ damage, especially to the liver and brain. Symptoms often mimic other conditions, making awareness of risk factors essential. Genetic testing and regular monitoring of copper levels can aid in early detection, ensuring that individuals receive the necessary treatment before significant damage occurs.

Once diagnosed, the focus shifts to ongoing management to prevent complications. This involves regular check-ups with healthcare providers who specialize in Wilson Disease. They can track copper levels, assess liver function, and adjust treatment plans accordingly. Proactive management through early diagnosis can lead to better health outcomes and improved quality of life.

Emphasis on Lifestyle Changes and Dietary Adjustments to Manage Symptoms Effectively

Lifestyle changes play a vital role in managing Wilson Disease symptoms and preventing copper accumulation in the body. This includes regular exercise, which can help maintain overall health and support liver function. Engaging in moderate physical activity such as walking, swimming, or yoga is beneficial. Additionally, avoiding alcohol and stress is essential, as both can exacerbate liver problems and other health issues associated with Wilson Disease.

Dietary adjustments are equally important for managing Wilson Disease. Individuals should avoid foods high in copper, such as shellfish, nuts, chocolate, and certain organ meats. Instead, focus on a balanced diet rich in fruits, vegetables, whole grains, and lean proteins. Consulting with a nutritionist experienced in Wilson Disease can provide personalized dietary guidance, ensuring that individuals receive the nutrients they need while minimizing copper intake. Regularly monitoring dietary choices helps in maintaining optimal health and managing symptoms effectively.

CHAPTER 1:

Overview of Wilson Disease

Description of Wilson Disease and Its Genetic Nature

Wilson Disease is a rare genetic disorder that affects copper metabolism in the body, leading to copper accumulation in tissues, particularly the liver, brain, and corneas. This accumulation can cause severe damage over time, affecting organ function and leading to life-threatening complications if not treated properly. Individuals with Wilson Disease typically inherit two copies of a mutated ATP7B gene, which is essential for regulating copper levels in the body.

Understanding Wilson Disease is crucial for early diagnosis and management. As a genetic condition, it can be passed down through families, making awareness of one's family history important for those with potential risk factors. This knowledge helps in proactive monitoring and early intervention to prevent severe complications associated with copper toxicity.

Explanation of the Role of ATP7B Gene Mutations

The ATP7B gene encodes a protein responsible for transporting copper into bile and helping excrete excess copper from the body. Mutations in this gene disrupt normal copper transport, resulting in impaired copper excretion and accumulation in organs. When the body cannot manage copper levels properly, it leads to cellular damage and various health issues, including liver disease and neurological problems.

To manage Wilson Disease effectively, it's essential to understand how these gene mutations affect copper metabolism. Individuals diagnosed with Wilson Disease should seek genetic counseling to understand the implications of ATP7B mutations on their health and the potential impact on family members. This understanding is crucial for making informed decisions regarding testing and treatment options.

Discussion on How Copper Accumulates in the Body

Copper accumulates in the body when there is a disruption in the normal process of copper absorption and excretion. In healthy individuals, copper is obtained from dietary sources and is excreted through bile. However, in those with Wilson Disease, the ATP7B gene mutations lead to insufficient excretion of copper, causing it to build up in organs over time. This accumulation can lead to oxidative stress and cell damage, particularly in the liver and brain.

Practical steps to monitor and manage copper levels include regular blood tests to assess copper levels and liver function. Those diagnosed with Wilson Disease should work closely with healthcare professionals to establish a management plan, including dietary restrictions and medication that help remove excess copper from the body.

Importance of Understanding Inheritance Patterns

Understanding the inheritance patterns of Wilson Disease is essential for affected families. Wilson Disease follows an autosomal recessive inheritance pattern, meaning a child must inherit two copies of the mutated gene—one from each parent—to develop the disease. Parents who are carriers (with one mutated copy) typically do not show symptoms but can pass the mutation to their children.

Families with a history of Wilson Disease should consider genetic testing and counseling to assess the risk of passing the disorder to future generations. This proactive approach allows for informed family planning and early intervention strategies for at-risk children, enabling them to be monitored for symptoms and receive timely treatment if necessary.

Common Demographics Affected by Wilson Disease

Wilson Disease affects individuals across various demographics, but it is most commonly diagnosed in children and young adults, typically between ages 5 and 35. The disease is more prevalent in certain populations, particularly those of Northern European descent. Awareness of demographic trends can help clinicians identify at-risk individuals and encourage testing in symptomatic cases.

Healthcare providers should remain vigilant for symptoms of Wilson Disease in patients who fit these demographics. Early detection through screening can lead to prompt treatment, which is essential for preventing organ damage and improving quality of life for affected individuals.

Statistics on Prevalence and Diagnosis Rates

Wilson Disease is estimated to affect approximately 1 in 30,000 individuals worldwide, but this number may vary depending on geographic and ethnic factors. Diagnosis rates can be low due to the overlapping symptoms with other conditions, leading to delays in treatment. On average, it takes several years for individuals to receive a correct diagnosis after the onset of symptoms.

To increase awareness and improve diagnosis rates, healthcare professionals must be educated on the symptoms and risk factors of Wilson Disease. Implementing routine screening for at-risk populations can also aid in the early identification of the disease, allowing for timely intervention and management.

Connection between Wilson Disease and Copper-Related Disorders

Wilson Disease is often associated with other copper-related disorders, such as Menkes disease, which is characterized by copper deficiency due to different genetic mutations. Both conditions illustrate the critical role copper plays in bodily functions, emphasizing the need for proper copper regulation. Understanding the connection between these disorders can provide insights into the importance of monitoring copper levels in patients with Wilson Disease.

To manage Wilson Disease effectively, individuals should be educated on the relationship between copper metabolism and overall health. Regular consultations with healthcare providers can help ensure that patients remain informed about their condition and any related disorders, promoting comprehensive care and management.

Importance of Genetic Testing and Family History

Genetic testing plays a crucial role in diagnosing Wilson Disease and identifying carriers within families. Testing for mutations in the ATP7B gene can confirm a diagnosis and allow for early interventions in at-risk individuals. Additionally, knowing family history is essential in assessing the likelihood of developing the disease and understanding potential health implications.

Individuals with a family history of Wilson Disease should seek genetic counseling to discuss testing options. By understanding their genetic risks, they can make informed decisions regarding lifestyle choices, monitoring strategies, and family planning, contributing to better long-term health outcomes.

Overview of the Disease Progression

Wilson Disease progresses through several stages, starting with asymptomatic copper accumulation and potentially leading to severe liver disease, neurological symptoms, and psychiatric issues if left untreated. Initially, symptoms may be subtle and nonspecific, such as fatigue or abdominal discomfort, making early diagnosis challenging. As the disease progresses, more serious complications can arise, including cirrhosis, hepatic failure, or neurological deficits.

Patients should be proactive in monitoring for symptoms and maintaining regular check-ups with healthcare providers to track disease progression. Early intervention, including medication and lifestyle changes, can significantly slow down or halt the progression of Wilson Disease, improving quality of life and reducing the risk of complications.

Symptoms Categorized by Age of Onset

Symptoms of Wilson Disease can vary based on the age of onset. In younger patients, symptoms often manifest as liver issues, such as jaundice or abdominal pain, while older individuals may experience neurological or psychiatric symptoms, such as tremors, mood changes, or cognitive decline. This variability can complicate diagnosis, as symptoms may be mistaken for other conditions.

To effectively manage symptoms, patients and families should be educated on the signs to watch for at different ages. Regular evaluations by healthcare professionals can help identify symptoms early, leading to prompt management strategies that address both liver health and neurological function.

Impact of Wilson Disease on Daily Life

Living with Wilson Disease can significantly impact daily life, requiring individuals to adhere to strict dietary modifications, regular medical check-ups, and possibly lifelong medication to manage copper levels. The psychological effects of managing a chronic condition can also be challenging, as individuals may experience anxiety related to symptoms or health complications.

To navigate these challenges, individuals should establish a routine that includes regular health monitoring and support networks. Connecting with support groups can provide emotional assistance and practical advice for managing daily life, ensuring that those affected by Wilson Disease can lead fulfilling lives while managing their condition.

Importance of Support Systems and Communities

Support systems and communities play a vital role in helping individuals cope with the challenges posed by Wilson Disease. These networks can provide emotional support, share experiences, and offer practical advice for managing symptoms and treatments. Many organizations and online communities focus on Wilson Disease awareness, fostering connections among those affected.

Engaging with support groups can also empower individuals to advocate for their health needs and stay informed about the latest research and treatment options. By participating in these communities, patients can enhance their coping strategies and access resources that improve their overall quality of life.

Introduction to Ongoing Research in Wilson Disease

Ongoing research in Wilson Disease focuses on understanding the mechanisms of copper metabolism and developing new treatments to enhance management strategies. Studies aim to improve early detection methods, explore gene therapy options, and evaluate the long-term effectiveness of existing therapies. This research is crucial for identifying innovative approaches to reduce the impact of copper accumulation on health.

Individuals with Wilson Disease and their families should stay informed about new developments in research. Engaging with healthcare providers about ongoing studies and clinical trials can provide opportunities for participation, helping to advance knowledge and treatment options for future patients.

CHAPTER 2:

Symptoms and Diagnosis

List of Early Symptoms

Wilson Disease can manifest through a range of early symptoms that may often be mistaken for other conditions. Common signs include fatigue, which can result in a lack of energy for daily activities, and jaundice, characterized by yellowing of the skin and eyes. These symptoms occur due to copper accumulation in the liver, impairing its function and leading to elevated bilirubin levels. Recognizing these initial signs is crucial for early intervention and management.

To monitor for these symptoms, individuals should maintain a log of any changes in energy levels, skin color, and overall well-being. Consulting a healthcare provider for a thorough evaluation is essential if these symptoms appear. Early detection can significantly improve outcomes, so understanding these signs can help individuals seek timely medical attention.

Discussion of Neurological Symptoms

As Wilson Disease progresses, neurological symptoms can emerge, impacting coordination and mental health. Common neurological signs include tremors, which can affect fine motor skills, and mood swings, leading to anxiety and depression. These symptoms arise due to copper buildup in the brain, disrupting normal brain function and leading to cognitive and motor impairments.

To manage these neurological symptoms, individuals are encouraged to engage in physical therapy and counseling, which can help improve motor skills and emotional well-being. Regular consultations with a neurologist can also aid in monitoring and adjusting treatment plans, ensuring that individuals receive comprehensive care tailored to their neurological needs.

Importance of Monitoring for Psychiatric Symptoms

Mental health monitoring is vital for individuals with Wilson Disease, as psychiatric symptoms can significantly affect quality of life. Symptoms may include depression, anxiety, and personality changes, which can be exacerbated by copper accumulation in the brain. Recognizing these signs early allows for prompt psychological intervention and support.

To effectively monitor psychiatric symptoms, individuals should maintain open communication with healthcare providers and family members about mood changes or emotional distress. Regular mental health assessments by a psychologist or psychiatrist can help develop effective coping strategies and therapeutic interventions tailored to the individual's needs.

How Symptoms Vary by Age and Severity

Wilson Disease symptoms can differ significantly based on an individual's age and the severity of copper accumulation. In younger individuals, liver-related symptoms may dominate, while older patients may present more pronounced neurological or psychiatric symptoms. This variability can complicate diagnosis and management, as symptoms can overlap with those of other conditions.

To adapt to these changes, healthcare providers should conduct age-appropriate assessments and tailor treatment plans accordingly. Regular follow-ups are crucial for monitoring symptom progression and adjusting interventions to align with the individual's evolving health status and needs.

Overview of Diagnostic Tests

Diagnostic tests play a critical role in identifying Wilson Disease and assessing copper levels in the body. Key tests include serum ceruloplasmin, which measures the protein responsible for copper transport in the blood. Low levels of ceruloplasmin can indicate copper accumulation, prompting further investigation.

In addition to serum ceruloplasmin testing, healthcare providers may recommend 24-hour urine copper tests to evaluate copper excretion. These tests provide valuable insights into the body's copper handling and help confirm a diagnosis, enabling timely and appropriate treatment interventions.

Role of Liver Biopsy in Confirming Diagnosis

A liver biopsy is often a definitive method for diagnosing Wilson Disease. During this procedure, a small sample of liver tissue is removed and examined for copper content and liver damage. This test helps confirm the diagnosis and assess the extent of liver damage caused by copper accumulation.

Individuals undergoing a liver biopsy should discuss the procedure with their healthcare provider, including the risks and benefits. Post-procedure care is essential to monitor for any complications and ensure a smooth recovery, facilitating timely diagnosis and treatment initiation.

Genetic Testing Options and Their Importance

Genetic testing for Wilson Disease is vital for confirming a diagnosis, especially in individuals with a family history of the disorder. Testing can identify mutations in the ATP7B gene, responsible for copper regulation in the body. A positive result can aid in early diagnosis, allowing for proactive management of the disease.

Families with a history of Wilson Disease should consider genetic counseling to understand the implications of testing. Genetic counselors can provide information on inheritance patterns, testing options, and potential outcomes, helping families make informed decisions about genetic testing and disease management.

Importance of Routine Screening for At-Risk Individuals

Routine screening is essential for individuals at risk of developing Wilson Disease, particularly those with a family history or symptoms. Early detection through regular blood tests and clinical evaluations can significantly improve management outcomes and prevent severe complications related to copper accumulation.

At-risk individuals should discuss screening options with their healthcare providers, who can recommend appropriate tests based on personal and family medical histories. Regular monitoring ensures that any emerging symptoms are addressed promptly, facilitating early intervention and ongoing health management.

How to Differentiate Between Wilson Disease and Other Liver Disorders

Differentiating Wilson Disease from other liver disorders can be challenging due to overlapping symptoms. Clinicians typically rely on a combination of clinical history, laboratory tests, and imaging studies to establish a clear diagnosis. Key differentiators include copper levels in the blood and urine and the presence of neurological symptoms.

To aid in diagnosis, individuals should provide comprehensive medical histories to their healthcare providers, detailing symptoms, family history, and lifestyle factors. This information is crucial for making accurate diagnoses and developing tailored treatment plans that address specific health concerns.

The Role of Clinical History in Diagnosis

Clinical history is a cornerstone of diagnosing Wilson Disease. A thorough assessment includes a review of symptoms, family history of genetic disorders, and any previous liver issues. This comprehensive approach helps healthcare providers identify patterns that may indicate Wilson Disease, guiding further testing and diagnosis.

Individuals should be proactive in discussing their medical histories with healthcare providers, highlighting any symptoms or family connections to liver disorders. This detailed history can streamline the diagnostic process, ensuring timely and appropriate interventions are implemented.

Importance of a Multidisciplinary Approach in Diagnosis

A multidisciplinary approach to diagnosing Wilson Disease is essential for comprehensive care. Involving specialists such as hepatologists, neurologists, and geneticists ensures that all aspects of the disease are addressed. This collaborative effort enhances the accuracy of diagnosis and the development of effective treatment plans.

Patients should seek healthcare providers who emphasize a team-based approach, ensuring access to various specialists. Regular case reviews and collaborative discussions among healthcare providers can optimize diagnosis and management strategies, leading to better patient outcomes.

Guidelines for Healthcare Providers

Healthcare providers are encouraged to follow established guidelines for diagnosing and managing Wilson Disease. These guidelines emphasize early identification through symptom recognition, appropriate laboratory testing, and a multidisciplinary approach. By adhering to these protocols, providers can improve diagnosis accuracy and treatment efficacy.

Healthcare providers should stay informed about the latest research and advancements in Wilson Disease management to enhance patient care. Continuous education and training can equip providers with the necessary tools and knowledge to effectively address the complexities of this rare genetic disorder.

Resources for Finding Specialists in Wilson Disease

Finding specialists in Wilson Disease can be challenging, but several resources are available to assist patients and families. Organizations such as the Wilson Disease Association provide directories of healthcare professionals specializing in this condition. These resources can help individuals connect with experts who understand the complexities of Wilson Disease.

Additionally, online support groups and forums can offer valuable recommendations for specialists and treatment centers. Engaging with others affected by Wilson Disease can provide insights and guidance on navigating the healthcare landscape, ensuring access to appropriate care and support.

CHAPTER 3:

Copper Accumulation and Liver Health

Explanation of Copper's Role in the Body

Copper is an essential trace mineral crucial for several bodily functions, including the formation of red blood cells, maintaining healthy bones and connective tissues, and supporting the immune system. It helps in the absorption of iron and plays a vital role in the functioning of enzymes involved in energy production and neurotransmitter synthesis. However, the body requires only a small amount of copper, and excess accumulation can lead to significant health issues.

To maintain a healthy balance, the liver typically regulates copper levels by excreting excess amounts into bile. In individuals with Wilson Disease, this regulatory process is disrupted due to a genetic mutation, leading to copper buildup. Understanding copper's essential role helps emphasize the importance of managing copper levels to prevent toxicity and maintain overall health.

Overview of Liver Function and Its Relation to Copper

The liver is a powerhouse organ responsible for detoxification, metabolism, and nutrient storage. It processes nutrients absorbed from the digestive tract and plays a key role in maintaining the body's overall balance, including regulating copper levels. The liver synthesizes proteins necessary for blood clotting and helps break down fats and carbohydrates, making it essential for energy production and storage.

In relation to copper, the liver absorbs and stores this mineral, releasing it as needed for bodily functions. However, when copper accumulation occurs, liver function can become impaired. This underscores the necessity of liver health in managing copper levels and preventing complications associated with Wilson Disease.

How Excess Copper Leads to Liver Damage

Excess copper in the body, particularly in the liver, can lead to cellular damage and inflammation, causing hepatocellular injury. Over time, this accumulation can result in liver fibrosis, where healthy liver tissue is replaced by scar tissue, impairing liver function. Elevated copper levels can disrupt the balance of other essential minerals, exacerbating liver damage and increasing the risk of cirrhosis.

To prevent liver damage, individuals with Wilson Disease must adhere to treatment regimens that reduce copper accumulation. This may include medications that promote copper excretion and dietary adjustments to limit copper intake. Understanding how excess copper leads to liver damage is essential for effective management and maintaining liver health.

Discussion of Liver Enzyme Tests and Their Significance

Liver enzyme tests are blood tests that measure the levels of enzymes released into the bloodstream when liver cells are damaged. Common tests include alanine aminotransferase (ALT) and Aspartate aminotransferase (AST). Elevated enzyme levels may indicate liver inflammation, damage, or dysfunction, which can be particularly relevant for those with Wilson Disease.

Regular monitoring of liver enzymes is crucial for assessing liver health and determining the effectiveness of treatment. A healthcare provider can interpret these test results to guide necessary adjustments in therapy or further diagnostic evaluations, ensuring proactive management of liver function.

Importance of Monitoring Liver Health Through Imaging

Imaging techniques, such as ultrasounds, CT scans, or MRIs, are essential tools for assessing liver health. These non-invasive methods help visualize liver structure and function, allowing healthcare providers to detect abnormalities such as lesions, fibrosis, or cirrhosis early. Regular imaging can provide crucial information about the progression of liver disease in individuals with Wilson Disease.

By incorporating imaging into routine care, healthcare providers can better monitor liver health and adjust treatment strategies as needed. This proactive approach can significantly impact long-term outcomes by identifying potential complications before they escalate.

Symptoms of Liver Dysfunction (e.g., Swelling, Pain)

Liver dysfunction may present with various symptoms, including abdominal swelling, pain, fatigue, jaundice (yellowing of the skin and eyes), and changes in appetite. Swelling may occur due to fluid retention (ascites) or liver enlargement, while pain can indicate inflammation or damage to liver tissues. Recognizing these symptoms early can lead to timely medical intervention.

If any signs of liver dysfunction arise, it is crucial to consult a healthcare professional for evaluation. Prompt attention to symptoms can prevent further damage and complications, emphasizing the importance of self-awareness and proactive health management for individuals with Wilson Disease.

Complications of Untreated Wilson Disease

Untreated Wilson Disease can lead to severe complications, including liver failure, neurological disorders, and psychiatric issues. As excess copper accumulates in the liver, it can cause cirrhosis, a condition characterized by irreversible liver scarring and loss of function. Additionally, copper buildup in the brain can result in movement disorders, cognitive decline, and mood disturbances.

Understanding these potential complications highlights the urgency of early diagnosis and treatment for Wilson Disease. Taking preventive measures can mitigate these risks and improve the overall quality of life for affected individuals.

Importance of Early Intervention for Liver Health

Early intervention is critical in managing Wilson Disease and preventing irreversible liver damage. Treatment options typically include medications that facilitate copper excretion, such as chelating agents or zinc supplements. Additionally, lifestyle modifications, such as dietary changes to limit copper intake, can significantly improve outcomes when implemented promptly.

Seeking medical advice as soon as Wilson Disease is suspected can lead to timely diagnosis and management. By prioritizing early intervention, individuals can effectively manage their condition and maintain better liver health.

Overview of Cirrhosis and Its Implications

Cirrhosis is a late-stage liver disease resulting from prolonged liver damage, leading to the replacement of healthy liver tissue with scar tissue. This condition can impair liver function significantly, affecting the body's ability to detoxify substances, produce essential proteins, and regulate various metabolic processes. Cirrhosis can be a life-threatening condition, emphasizing the need for preventive measures in those with Wilson Disease.

Management of cirrhosis often requires lifestyle changes, regular monitoring, and in severe cases, liver transplantation. Understanding the implications of cirrhosis underlines the importance of early detection and intervention in managing Wilson Disease to prevent the progression of liver damage.

Discussion on Liver Transplantation as a Treatment Option

Liver transplantation may be considered for individuals with Wilson Disease who develop severe liver damage or cirrhosis and do not respond to other treatments. This surgical procedure involves replacing the diseased liver with a healthy donor liver, offering a potential cure for the underlying condition. It is essential to thoroughly evaluate candidates for transplantation to ensure they are suitable for the procedure.

Post-transplant care is crucial, as recipients must adhere to strict medication regimens to prevent organ rejection and monitor liver function closely. Understanding the transplantation process and its implications can help individuals with advanced Wilson Disease consider this option as a viable treatment pathway.

Importance of Regular Check-Ups for Liver Function

Regular check-ups are vital for monitoring liver function in individuals with Wilson Disease. These appointments typically involve blood tests to assess liver enzymes and overall health, allowing healthcare providers to track any changes over time. Routine check-ups facilitate early detection of potential complications and ensure timely adjustments to treatment plans as necessary.

Establishing a consistent follow-up schedule with healthcare providers fosters proactive management of liver health. By prioritizing regular check-ups, individuals can maintain optimal liver function and mitigate the risks associated with Wilson Disease.

Role of Lifestyle Modifications in Maintaining Liver Health

Lifestyle modifications play a crucial role in maintaining liver health for individuals with Wilson Disease. This includes adhering to a copper-restricted diet, avoiding alcohol, engaging in regular exercise, and managing weight to reduce strain on the liver. Implementing these changes can significantly improve overall health and support the liver's ability to process and eliminate excess copper.

Education about the impact of lifestyle choices empowers individuals to take control of their health. By making informed decisions and prioritizing liver-friendly habits, individuals can enhance their well-being and minimize complications associated with Wilson Disease.

Research on Liver Health Outcomes in Wilson Disease Patients

Ongoing research into liver health outcomes for individuals with Wilson Disease is essential for advancing understanding and treatment options. Studies aim to explore the efficacy of various treatment modalities, the long-term impacts of lifestyle changes, and the relationship between early intervention and liver health outcomes. This research is crucial for developing evidence-based guidelines for managing Wilson Disease effectively.

Staying informed about current research can help individuals and healthcare providers make informed decisions regarding treatment options and lifestyle modifications. Engaging with emerging findings fosters a proactive approach to managing Wilson Disease and optimizing liver health outcomes.

CHAPTER 4:

Treatment Options

Overview of Chelation Therapy and Its Purpose

Chelation therapy is a medical procedure used to remove excess copper from the body, particularly in patients with Wilson disease. The therapy works by administering chelating agents that bind to copper, allowing it to be excreted through the urine. This helps prevent further accumulation of copper in organs, especially the liver and brain, and can significantly improve overall health and quality of life.

For those newly diagnosed, understanding chelation therapy is crucial. It involves regular visits to a healthcare provider who will administer the treatment and monitor progress. Patients should be aware of the importance of following the prescribed chelation regimen closely to effectively manage their copper levels and reduce the risk of organ damage.

Description of Common Chelating Agents

The most commonly used chelating agent for Wilson disease is penicillamine, which binds to copper in the bloodstream and promotes its excretion. Other agents include trientine and zinc, which also play roles in managing copper levels. Each agent has its specific dosing, administration methods, and indications, making it essential for patients to work closely with their healthcare team to determine the best option.

When starting treatment, it's important for patients to educate themselves on how these agents function and their expected outcomes. This knowledge can empower patients in discussions with their doctors about their treatment plan and help them understand any adjustments that may be needed over time.

Explanation of the Timing and Method of Chelation Therapy

Chelation therapy typically begins after a definitive diagnosis of Wilson disease, and the timing is crucial. Treatments usually start when liver copper levels are high or when symptoms appear. Penicillamine is usually administered orally, and it's essential to adhere to the prescribed schedule, which may be daily or multiple times a week depending on the severity of copper accumulation.

Patients should ensure they understand how to take their medication correctly—whether on an empty stomach or with food—and should not skip doses. Regular follow-ups are necessary to assess copper levels and adjust treatment as needed to maintain effective control over the condition.

Potential Side Effects of Chelation Therapy

While chelation therapy is effective, it can have side effects, including gastrointestinal issues, rashes, and potential kidney problems. These side effects vary from person to person, and it's crucial for patients to report any adverse reactions to their healthcare provider immediately.

Patients should be prepared to manage side effects by maintaining good communication with their healthcare team. They can also benefit from support groups where they can share experiences and tips on how to cope with side effects while continuing treatment effectively.

Role of Zinc Therapy in Managing Copper Levels

Zinc therapy serves as an alternative or adjunct treatment for managing copper levels in Wilson disease. Zinc helps to block copper absorption in the intestines and promotes the excretion of copper already present in the body. This can be particularly beneficial for patients who may not tolerate other chelating agents well.

To implement zinc therapy, patients should consult their healthcare provider to determine the appropriate dosage and timing. Regular monitoring of zinc levels is also necessary to avoid potential deficiencies, as excess zinc can interfere with the absorption of other essential minerals.

Importance of Regular Monitoring During Treatment

Regular monitoring is critical in managing Wilson disease effectively. Healthcare providers typically schedule routine blood tests to measure copper and liver enzyme levels, helping to assess how well treatment is working. Monitoring also allows for timely adjustments to the treatment plan, minimizing the risk of complications.

Patients should actively participate in their monitoring process by keeping a log of their test results and any symptoms they experience. This information can help facilitate productive conversations with healthcare providers, leading to more tailored and effective treatment strategies.

Discussion on Liver Transplantation as a Last Resort

In severe cases of Wilson disease, when liver damage is extensive and other treatments have failed, liver transplantation may be considered a last resort. This option is typically explored when a patient's liver function declines significantly or when they develop life-threatening complications related to copper overload.

Patients and families should be informed about the liver transplant process, including donor matching, the surgical procedure, and the post-operative care required. Engaging with a transplant center early can provide valuable information and support throughout the evaluation and potential transplantation process.

Supportive Care for Managing Symptoms

Supportive care is essential for managing symptoms of Wilson disease alongside medical treatment. This may include physical therapy, counseling, and nutritional support to help address the physical and emotional challenges that arise from the condition. Engaging in regular exercise and maintaining a balanced diet can also contribute to overall well-being.

Patients should actively seek out resources and support groups that provide information and community connections. Sharing experiences with others facing similar challenges can help patients feel less isolated and more empowered in managing their condition.

Importance of Adherence to Treatment Plans

Adherence to treatment plans is vital for individuals with Wilson disease to prevent copper accumulation and associated complications. Patients should prioritize taking medications as prescribed and attending regular follow-up appointments to monitor their health status. Consistency in treatment can lead to improved outcomes and a better quality of life.

To stay on track, patients can utilize medication reminders, keep a daily journal, or enlist the help of family members to ensure they are following their treatment regimen closely. Establishing a routine can also help make adherence easier and more manageable.

Potential Interactions with Other Medications

Patients with Wilson disease should be aware of potential interactions between their chelation therapy and other medications they may be taking. Some drugs can affect the absorption and effectiveness of chelating agents, while others may exacerbate side effects. Therefore, it's crucial to provide a comprehensive list of all medications to healthcare providers.

Before starting any new medications, including over-the-counter products or supplements, patients should consult with their doctor. This proactive approach helps prevent complications and ensures that all aspects of treatment work harmoniously.

Role of Clinical Trials in Exploring New Treatments

Clinical trials play a significant role in advancing treatment options for Wilson disease. Participating in clinical trials can provide patients access to innovative therapies and contribute to the development of new treatment protocols. Researchers often look for volunteers who meet specific criteria, making it essential for patients to understand the requirements and potential benefits of participation.

Patients interested in clinical trials should discuss this option with their healthcare provider. They can also seek information from organizations dedicated to Wilson disease to find ongoing studies that align with their treatment goals and health status.

Patient Stories and Testimonials on Treatment Experiences

Patient stories and testimonials can be powerful sources of information and inspiration for individuals managing Wilson disease. Hearing firsthand experiences can provide insights into the challenges faced and the coping strategies employed, offering hope and encouragement for those starting their treatment journey.

Patients should actively seek out these stories through support groups, online forums, or healthcare provider recommendations. Sharing their experiences can also foster a sense of community and support, making the journey through treatment feel less daunting.

Resources for Finding Treatment Centers

Finding specialized treatment centers for Wilson disease is crucial for effective management of the condition. Patients should consult their healthcare providers for referrals to liver specialists or clinics with expertise in genetic disorders. Additionally, organizations focused on Wilson disease often have directories of qualified treatment centers.

Exploring online resources can also help locate nearby facilities. Patients should prioritize seeking treatment from centers that provide comprehensive care, including access to nutritionists, mental health professionals, and support groups to address all aspects of living with Wilson disease.

CHAPTER 5:

Dietary Adjustments

Importance of Dietary Changes in Managing Wilson Disease

Dietary changes play a crucial role in managing Wilson Disease, as they help control copper accumulation in the body. By avoiding high-copper foods and incorporating low-copper options, individuals can significantly reduce their copper intake, ultimately preventing organ damage, especially to the liver. Consistent adherence to these dietary changes is essential for maintaining overall health and well-being.

Implementing dietary changes also means being proactive about meal planning and preparation. Individuals and families must educate themselves on suitable food choices and develop a meal plan that reflects these choices. This way, they can enjoy a varied diet while managing their condition effectively.

List of Foods High in Copper to Avoid (e.g., Shellfish, Nuts)

Certain foods are particularly high in copper and should be avoided by individuals with Wilson Disease. Shellfish, organ meats, nuts, seeds, and chocolate are prime examples of foods that can contribute to excessive copper levels. By avoiding these items, patients can reduce their risk of copper buildup in the body.

To make informed decisions, individuals should familiarize themselves with specific foods high in copper. This knowledge helps them navigate grocery shopping and meal planning more effectively, ensuring they stick to their dietary restrictions without feeling deprived.

Recommended Foods for a Low-Copper Diet

A low-copper diet includes a variety of foods that help minimize copper intake. Recommended options include most fruits and vegetables, grains like rice and pasta, and certain dairy products. These foods not only provide essential nutrients but also help maintain a balanced diet while keeping copper levels low.

Incorporating these low-copper foods into daily meals is essential for effective management. Patients should focus on fresh, whole foods while being mindful of their copper content, ensuring they maintain a healthy diet without compromising their health.

Importance of Hydration and Balanced Nutrition

Staying hydrated is vital for individuals with Wilson Disease, as it supports liver function and overall health. Drinking plenty of water throughout the day helps flush out toxins and maintain proper bodily functions. A balanced diet that includes appropriate portions of carbohydrates, proteins, and fats also supports overall nutrition and wellness.

Proper hydration and balanced nutrition work together to promote optimal health in patients. By prioritizing water intake and balanced meals, individuals can enhance their body's ability to cope with the effects of Wilson Disease and reduce the risk of complications.

Role of a Dietitian in Meal Planning

A registered dietitian plays a key role in managing Wilson Disease through personalized meal planning. They can help create an individualized dietary plan that aligns with the patient's preferences, nutritional needs, and copper restrictions. This expert guidance is essential for navigating the complexities of dietary changes.

Working with a dietitian allows patients to receive tailored support, including recipe ideas and meal prep strategies. This collaboration can empower individuals and families to make informed food choices that adhere to dietary restrictions while maintaining a satisfying and varied diet.

Understanding Food Labels and Hidden Copper Sources

Understanding food labels is crucial for individuals managing Wilson Disease. Many packaged foods may contain hidden copper sources, such as additives and preservatives. By learning to read labels carefully, patients can identify and avoid foods that could contribute to copper buildup.

Hidden sources of copper can also be found in foods that may not be initially obvious. Patients should be vigilant about researching unfamiliar ingredients and seeking out resources that provide information on hidden copper sources in various foods.

Importance of Supplements and Vitamins

Supplements and vitamins may be necessary for individuals with Wilson Disease to ensure they receive essential nutrients while adhering to a low-copper diet. Vitamin E, for example, can help protect liver health, while vitamin D supports bone health. It's important to consult a healthcare provider before starting any supplementation regimen.

Incorporating the right supplements can help address potential nutrient deficiencies that arise from dietary restrictions. Regular check-ups with a healthcare provider can ensure that the supplements taken align with individual health needs and support overall wellness.

Discussion on the Impact of Alcohol on Liver Health

Alcohol consumption poses significant risks for individuals with Wilson Disease due to its detrimental effects on liver health. Alcohol can exacerbate liver damage and interfere with the body's ability to process copper effectively. Therefore, it is generally recommended that individuals with Wilson Disease abstain from alcohol altogether.

Educating oneself about the impact of alcohol on liver health is essential for managing the condition.

Individuals should be aware of alternative beverages and strategies for social situations that do not involve alcohol consumption, ensuring they protect their liver health.

Meal Planning Tips for Families

Meal planning can be a collaborative effort for families managing Wilson Disease. Involving all family members in meal preparation fosters understanding and adherence to dietary restrictions. Creating a weekly meal plan that includes low-copper foods helps everyone stay on track and makes mealtime more enjoyable.

In addition, families can share recipes and cooking responsibilities, making the process of meal planning a fun and inclusive activity. This collaboration not only supports dietary adherence but also strengthens family bonds as they work together to manage health challenges.

Cooking Methods That Reduce Copper Absorption

Certain cooking methods can help reduce copper absorption in foods. Boiling vegetables, for example, can leach some copper into the water, which is then discarded. Steaming, baking, or grilling foods are also effective methods that can help minimize copper content while retaining nutritional value.

Using these cooking techniques allows individuals to enjoy a variety of dishes without excessive copper intake. Experimenting with different cooking methods can lead to discovering new and enjoyable low-copper recipes that fit within dietary guidelines.

Importance of Family Support in Dietary Adherence

Family support is crucial for individuals managing Wilson Disease and adhering to dietary changes. Encouragement from family members can significantly impact a patient's commitment to maintaining their dietary restrictions. A supportive environment fosters adherence and can lead to better health outcomes.

Families can play an active role by learning about Wilson Disease and its dietary implications. This shared knowledge helps create a supportive atmosphere where family members can encourage healthy eating habits and participate in meal preparation together.

Patient Resources for Dietary Education

Numerous resources are available for patients seeking dietary education on managing Wilson Disease. Organizations dedicated to liver health and genetic disorders often provide informative materials, support groups, and online forums where individuals can share experiences and strategies.

Accessing these resources can empower patients to make informed dietary choices and connect with others facing similar challenges. Utilizing educational materials ensures that individuals have the necessary knowledge to manage their condition effectively.

Tips for Dining Out While Managing Wilson Disease

Dining out can be challenging for individuals managing Wilson Disease, but with some planning, it can be enjoyable. Prior to visiting a restaurant, patients should research menus online to identify low-copper options and don't hesitate to ask restaurant staff about ingredients and preparation methods.

When dining out, it's helpful to communicate dietary restrictions clearly to ensure safe meal choices. Making informed decisions and advocating for one's health allows individuals to enjoy social dining experiences while adhering to their dietary needs.

CHAPTER 6:

Lifestyle Changes for Management

Importance of Regular Medical Check-Ups

Regular medical check-ups are crucial for individuals with Wilson Disease, as they allow for continuous monitoring of copper levels and liver function. During these visits, healthcare providers can perform blood tests and liver function tests to assess the effectiveness of treatment and make necessary adjustments. It's recommended to schedule these check-ups every three to six months, depending on the individual's condition.

In addition to monitoring physical health, regular appointments provide a platform for discussing any new symptoms or concerns with a healthcare professional. Establishing a good relationship with a physician who understands Wilson Disease can ensure that patients receive tailored advice and interventions to prevent complications. Always keep a record of symptoms and questions to discuss during appointments for effective communication.

Overview of Stress Management Techniques

Stress management is vital for individuals with Wilson Disease, as stress can exacerbate symptoms and affect overall well-being. Techniques such as mindfulness, meditation, and deep-breathing exercises can help reduce stress levels. Practicing mindfulness involves focusing on the present moment, which can be achieved through activities like yoga or guided meditation sessions. These techniques not only lower stress but also promote a sense of calm and improve mental clarity.

Incorporating stress-relief activities into daily routines can be beneficial. Consider setting aside time each day for mindfulness practices, whether it's a few minutes of meditation in the morning or a longer yoga session in the evening. Additionally, engaging in hobbies that bring joy can also help manage stress levels and provide an outlet for emotions.

Role of Exercise in Overall Health

Exercise plays a significant role in maintaining overall health and managing Wilson Disease. Regular physical activity helps improve liver function, enhance mood, and increase energy levels. Aim for at least 150 minutes of moderate-intensity exercise each week, which can include activities like walking, swimming, or cycling. Start with small, achievable goals, and gradually increase intensity and duration as fitness levels improve.

Incorporating strength training exercises at least twice a week can also be beneficial. Resistance exercises help maintain muscle mass, which is particularly important for those with Wilson Disease who may experience fatigue or weakness. Always consult a healthcare provider before starting a new exercise regimen to ensure safety and appropriateness based on individual health conditions.

Importance of Sleep Hygiene and Routines

Establishing good sleep hygiene is essential for individuals with Wilson Disease, as adequate rest supports overall health and helps manage symptoms. Aim for 7-9 hours of quality sleep each night. Create a consistent bedtime routine by going to bed and waking up at the same time every day, even on weekends. This routine signals the body when it's time to sleep and helps regulate the sleep-wake cycle.

Additionally, consider the sleep environment. Ensure the bedroom is dark, cool, and quiet to promote restful sleep. Limiting screen time before bed and avoiding caffeine or heavy meals in the evening can also improve sleep quality. If sleep disturbances persist, consult a healthcare professional for further evaluation and support.

Discussion on Avoiding Environmental Toxins

Avoiding environmental toxins is vital for individuals with Wilson Disease, as exposure can exacerbate symptoms and further damage the liver. Start by identifying common sources of toxins in everyday life, such as household cleaning products, pesticides, and heavy metals. Opt for natural, non-toxic alternatives when possible, and ensure proper ventilation when using chemicals in the home.

Furthermore, being mindful of dietary choices can help reduce toxin intake. Choose organic fruits and vegetables when available to minimize exposure to pesticides. Regularly check local advisories for safe water and fish consumption, especially if living near polluted areas. Staying informed about potential toxins in the environment can empower individuals to make healthier choices.

Importance of Staying Hydrated

Staying hydrated is crucial for individuals with Wilson Disease, as proper hydration aids in detoxifying the body and supports liver function. Aim to drink at least eight 8-ounce glasses of water daily, or more depending on activity levels and climate. Keep a reusable water bottle handy as a reminder to drink throughout the day.

In addition to water, consider incorporating hydrating foods into your diet, such as fruits and vegetables with high water content, like cucumbers, oranges, and watermelon. Monitoring urine color can also be an effective way to assess hydration levels; aim for light yellow urine, indicating proper hydration. If you experience symptoms like fatigue or dizziness, increase fluid intake immediately

Role of Social Support in Managing Chronic Illness

Social support is an essential component of managing Wilson Disease, as it helps alleviate feelings of isolation and provides emotional comfort. Connecting with friends, family, and support groups can foster a sense of community and belonging. Consider joining local or online support groups specifically for individuals with Wilson Disease to share experiences, challenges, and coping strategies.

Engaging in open communication with loved ones about your condition can also strengthen these relationships. Sharing information about Wilson Disease helps them understand your needs and concerns better, allowing for more meaningful support. Don't hesitate to lean on your support network, as having people to talk to can significantly enhance emotional well-being.

Tips for Managing Work and School Life

Managing work and school life with Wilson Disease requires effective planning and communication. Prioritize tasks by creating a daily schedule that allows for breaks and flexibility. Use tools like planners or digital apps to keep track of deadlines and appointments, ensuring that health needs are integrated into your routine.

Additionally, consider discussing your condition with employers or educators to seek accommodations that can support your health. This may include flexible work hours, the option to work from home, or adjustments in workload. Being proactive about your health in professional and academic settings can help create a supportive environment conducive to both personal and career success.

Importance of Keeping a Health Journal

Keeping a health journal is an effective strategy for managing Wilson Disease and tracking symptoms, treatments, and lifestyle changes. Document daily experiences, including physical symptoms, emotional well-being, and dietary habits. This practice helps identify patterns that may influence symptoms and informs discussions with healthcare providers.

Incorporate sections in the journal for medication schedules, medical appointments, and test results to maintain comprehensive records of health status. Review the journal regularly to reflect on progress and make necessary adjustments to your management plan. A health journal empowers individuals to take an active role in their care and enhances communication with healthcare professionals.

Strategies for Staying Informed About Wilson Disease

Staying informed about Wilson Disease is crucial for effective management and empowerment. Begin by accessing reputable sources, such as healthcare organizations, academic articles, and patient advocacy groups. Subscribing to newsletters or following online forums can provide updates on research, treatment options, and community events.

Engaging in educational opportunities, such as webinars or workshops focused on Wilson Disease, can enhance understanding and provide valuable insights. Encourage discussions with healthcare providers to clarify any questions or concerns, ensuring that information is current and tailored to individual health needs. Knowledge is a powerful tool in navigating the complexities of living with Wilson Disease.

Importance of Community Resources and Support Groups

Community resources and support groups play a vital role in providing assistance and encouragement for those living with Wilson Disease. Local hospitals, health clinics, and nonprofit organizations often offer programs, workshops, and resources tailored to individuals with chronic illnesses. Research and reach out to these resources to explore available services, including counseling, nutritional support, and financial assistance.

Joining support groups, either in-person or online, creates opportunities to connect with others facing similar challenges. These groups provide a platform for sharing experiences, learning coping strategies, and fostering friendships. Participating in community events related to Wilson Disease can enhance social connections and contribute to a sense of belonging.

Engaging in Hobbies and Activities for Mental Health

Engaging in hobbies and activities is essential for maintaining mental health while managing Wilson Disease. Find enjoyable activities that promote relaxation and creativity, such as painting, gardening, or playing a musical instrument. Allocating time for these pursuits can serve as a positive distraction and boost overall well-being.

Consider exploring new interests or skills that promote social interaction, such as joining a book club or a local sports team. Participating in group activities fosters connections with others and helps combat feelings of isolation. Incorporating hobbies into daily life not only enhances mental health but also enriches personal fulfillment and joy.

Patient Stories on Lifestyle Transformations

Patient stories provide valuable insights and inspiration for individuals managing Wilson Disease. Listening to the experiences of others who have successfully navigated lifestyle changes can offer practical tips and encouragement. Look for testimonials through support groups, blogs, or social media platforms where individuals share their journeys and transformations.

These stories often highlight the importance of proactive health management, including dietary adjustments, exercise routines, and emotional support. Learning from the experiences of others can empower individuals to make informed decisions about their health and inspire a sense of hope for positive changes in their own lives.

CHAPTER 7:

Coping Mechanisms

Importance of Mental Health Awareness in Chronic Illness

Mental health is a critical aspect of managing chronic illnesses like Wilson Disease. Awareness can help patients recognize that emotional well-being is as important as physical health. This understanding encourages individuals to prioritize their mental health, fostering a holistic approach to treatment and recovery.

By acknowledging the impact of chronic illness on mental health, patients can engage in proactive measures such as mindfulness, self-care practices, and seeking professional help. Recognizing the signs of mental distress can also lead to earlier intervention, ultimately improving quality of life and overall health outcomes.

Overview of Common Emotional Responses to Diagnosis

Receiving a diagnosis of Wilson Disease can evoke a range of emotional responses, including shock, fear, anger, and sadness. These feelings are normal and part of the coping process. Understanding that these emotions are common can provide reassurance and normalize the experience for patients and their families.

Moreover, it's essential to recognize that individuals may experience these emotions differently and at varying intensities. Accepting these feelings as part of the journey can help patients navigate their emotional landscape more effectively, allowing them to seek support when needed.

Strategies for Dealing with Anxiety and Depression

To cope with anxiety and depression, individuals can employ practical strategies such as mindfulness exercises, deep breathing, and physical activity.

Engaging in regular exercise not only boosts mood but also helps manage stress levels. Establishing a daily routine can also provide structure and a sense of control, which is particularly beneficial for individuals facing chronic illness.

Additionally, journaling can be an effective tool for processing emotions and reflecting on daily experiences. Setting aside time each day to write about feelings or challenges can enhance self-awareness and foster a sense of accomplishment, which is crucial for mental well-being.

Importance of Therapy and Counseling

Therapy and counseling offer invaluable support for individuals coping with the emotional toll of chronic illnesses. A trained mental health professional can provide coping strategies tailored to each patient's unique situation, helping them navigate their feelings and develop resilience.

Furthermore, therapy can facilitate communication about the challenges of living with Wilson Disease. Whether through individual therapy or family counseling, these sessions can foster understanding and support among loved ones, creating a more supportive home environment.

Role of Support Groups in Coping

Support groups provide a safe space for individuals with Wilson Disease to share experiences and feelings. Connecting with others facing similar challenges can reduce feelings of isolation and promote a sense of community. This shared understanding fosters camaraderie, encouragement, and the exchange of practical coping strategies.

Participating in a support group can also enhance emotional resilience. Listening to others' journeys can offer new perspectives, reinforce hope, and motivate individuals to adopt positive coping mechanisms, ultimately improving their quality of life.

Discussion on Communication with Family and Friends

Effective communication with family and friends is vital for maintaining strong support systems. Being open about one's diagnosis, treatment, and emotional challenges fosters understanding and reduces misunderstandings. Patients should aim to express their needs clearly, ensuring that loved ones know how best to provide support.

Additionally, involving family and friends in the education process about Wilson Disease can create a shared commitment to managing the illness. Providing them with resources or inviting them to attend medical appointments can help them better understand the condition and its implications, promoting empathy and informed support.

Strategies for Educating Loved Ones about Wilson Disease

Educating loved ones about Wilson Disease can significantly improve the support system for patients. Begin by sharing reliable resources, such as brochures or reputable websites that outline the condition, its symptoms, and its management. This foundational knowledge helps dispel myths and misconceptions, fostering a more informed environment.

Encouraging open discussions can further enhance understanding. Patients can invite their loved ones to ask questions and share their feelings about the diagnosis, which can help address concerns and solidify support. A well-informed support network can be instrumental in navigating the challenges of chronic illness.

Importance of Setting Realistic Health Goals

Setting realistic health goals is essential for maintaining motivation and a sense of achievement. Patients should start by identifying specific, measurable, attainable, relevant, and time-bound (SMART) goals related to their health and well-being. This structured approach provides clarity and focus, making it easier to track progress.

Regularly reviewing and adjusting these goals ensures they remain relevant and achievable. Celebrating small victories along the way can enhance motivation and reinforce positive behaviors, contributing to improved health outcomes over time.

Techniques for Self-Advocacy in Healthcare

Self-advocacy is crucial for effectively managing health care in chronic illness. Patients can begin by preparing for medical appointments with a list of questions and concerns. This preparation empowers them to engage actively in discussions with healthcare providers, ensuring their voices are heard.

Additionally, keeping detailed records of symptoms, medications, and treatment responses can facilitate more informed conversations with healthcare professionals. This proactive approach enables patients to take charge of their health care, leading to better outcomes and satisfaction with their treatment.

Resources for Mental Health Support

Numerous resources are available for mental health support, ranging from online platforms to local organizations. Patients can explore mental health hotlines, therapy apps, and community resources that provide counseling and support groups. These tools can offer immediate assistance and connection to professionals who understand the challenges of chronic illness.

Furthermore, many organizations dedicated to specific conditions, such as Wilson Disease, provide tailored resources, including educational materials, workshops, and online forums. Leveraging these resources can help individuals find the support they need to navigate their mental health challenges effectively.

Importance of Humor and Positivity

Maintaining a sense of humor and positivity can significantly impact coping with chronic illness. Engaging in activities that bring joy, such as watching comedies or spending time with uplifting friends, can help alleviate stress and improve mood. Humor serves as a powerful tool for perspective, allowing individuals to find lightness even in challenging circumstances.

Additionally, practicing gratitude by acknowledging positive aspects of life can shift focus away from illness-related difficulties. Keeping a gratitude journal or sharing positive experiences with loved ones can cultivate a more optimistic outlook, which is essential for overall well-being.

Stories of Resilience from Wilson Disease Patients

Listening to stories of resilience from other Wilson Disease patients can provide inspiration and hope. These narratives often highlight the triumphs over adversity, showcasing how individuals have navigated the challenges of the disease while finding ways to thrive. Personal accounts can serve as powerful motivators, demonstrating that it's possible to live a fulfilling life despite chronic illness.

Moreover, sharing one's own story can empower others facing similar struggles. By discussing personal experiences and coping strategies, individuals can foster a sense of community and connection, encouraging mutual support and resilience in the face of Wilson Disease.

Encouragement for Seeking Help When Needed

It's essential for individuals coping with Wilson Disease to recognize when they need help and to seek it. This may include reaching out to healthcare professionals, mental health counselors, or support groups. Acknowledging the need for assistance is a strength, not a weakness, and can significantly improve one's quality of life.

Encouragement should extend to families and friends as well. Supporting loved ones in seeking help and being an active participant in their journey can make a profound difference. Whether through attending therapy sessions together or engaging in open discussions, fostering a culture of seeking help can lead to healthier, more resilient individuals

CHAPTER 8:

Managing Complications

Overview of Potential Complications (e.g., Neurological Damage)

Wilson disease can lead to various complications, especially if left untreated, with neurological damage being one of the most serious. Excess copper can accumulate in the brain, potentially causing cognitive decline, personality changes, tremors, and motor control issues. Recognizing these risks is vital for early intervention, as neurological complications can significantly impact quality of life.

To prevent neurological damage, patients should work closely with their healthcare providers to monitor their copper levels and adjust treatment as necessary. Regular check-ups can help detect any early signs of neurological complications, allowing for prompt treatment and better outcomes. Maintaining open communication with healthcare professionals is essential to ensure all potential complications are addressed effectively.

Importance of Regular Neurological Evaluations

Regular neurological evaluations are crucial for individuals with Wilson disease, as they help assess cognitive function and motor skills over time. These evaluations can identify any changes or declines in neurological health early on, enabling timely interventions that can prevent or mitigate damage. By scheduling these assessments at least once a year, patients can keep their healthcare providers informed about their neurological status.

Patients and caregivers should prepare for these evaluations by documenting any changes in behavior, mood, or motor function. This information can provide valuable insights to healthcare providers, making it easier to tailor treatment plans and adjust medications as necessary. Collaborating with neurologists can ensure a comprehensive approach to managing Wilson disease effectively.

Strategies for Managing Medication Side Effects

Managing medication side effects is an important aspect of Wilson disease treatment, as medications like chelators can lead to gastrointestinal issues, fatigue, or other symptoms. Patients should discuss potential side effects with their healthcare providers and develop a plan to manage them effectively. This may include taking medications with food, adjusting doses, or switching to alternative therapies if necessary.

In addition, patients can benefit from maintaining a side effects journal, tracking symptoms, and their severity. This record will help healthcare providers make informed decisions about treatment adjustments, enhancing patient comfort and adherence to medication regimens.

Importance of Recognizing Warning Signs of Complications

Recognizing the warning signs of complications is crucial for individuals with Wilson disease to prevent serious health issues. Common symptoms indicating potential complications include severe headaches, sudden changes in behavior, unusual tremors, or difficulty with coordination. Awareness of these signs empowers patients and caregivers to act quickly and seek medical attention.

Educating patients and their families about these warning signs can lead to timely interventions and better outcomes. Establishing a clear plan of action for when symptoms arise, including contact information for healthcare providers and emergency services, can significantly enhance patient safety and health management.

Role of Specialists in Managing Complications

Specialists play a vital role in managing complications associated with Wilson disease. A multidisciplinary approach, including hepatologists, neurologists, dietitians, and mental health professionals, can provide comprehensive care tailored to individual needs. Regular consultations with these specialists ensure that all aspects of the disease are addressed, minimizing the risk of complications.

Patients should actively seek referrals to specialists as part of their care plan. Coordinating care between various healthcare providers helps create a holistic treatment approach, leading to better management of symptoms and complications associated with Wilson disease.

Overview of Emergency Protocols for Severe Symptoms

Having a clear understanding of emergency protocols for severe symptoms is essential for individuals with Wilson disease. In situations such as sudden confusion, extreme fatigue, or seizures, patients should know when to seek immediate medical attention. Developing a personalized emergency action plan that outlines specific symptoms requiring urgent care can significantly improve outcomes during crises.

Patients and caregivers should keep a list of emergency contacts, including healthcare providers, poison control, and local hospitals. Familiarizing oneself with the nearest emergency room and its protocols for handling Wilson disease complications can reduce anxiety during emergencies and ensure timely intervention when needed.

Importance of Maintaining a Symptom Diary

Maintaining a symptom diary can be a powerful tool for managing Wilson disease. By recording daily symptoms, medication adherence, and any dietary changes, patients can identify patterns and triggers that may affect their health. This diary not only helps patients communicate effectively with their healthcare providers but also aids in personalizing treatment plans.

To create an effective symptom diary, patients should document their symptoms at the same time each day and include details such as severity and duration. Regularly reviewing this diary with healthcare professionals can enhance understanding of the disease and lead to better management strategies tailored to individual needs.

Strategies for Navigating Healthcare Systems

Navigating healthcare systems can be challenging for individuals with Wilson disease, but there are strategies to make the process smoother. Patients should establish a primary care provider who understands Wilson disease and can coordinate referrals to specialists as needed. Keeping organized medical records and a list of questions for appointments can help ensure comprehensive care.

Additionally, patients can benefit from engaging with patient advocacy organizations that provide resources and support for navigating the healthcare system. These organizations often offer guidance on insurance issues, access to specialists, and community resources, empowering patients to take control of their healthcare journey.

Patient Advocacy in Addressing Complications

Patient advocacy is crucial in addressing complications associated with Wilson disease. Patients should feel empowered to communicate openly with their healthcare providers about their concerns, symptoms, and treatment options. Engaging in discussions about care preferences and treatment plans can lead to more personalized and effective management strategies.

Joining support groups or online communities can also enhance advocacy efforts. Sharing experiences and learning from others can provide valuable insights into managing complications and navigating healthcare challenges, fostering a sense of community and support among patients.

Importance of Continuous Education on Wilson Disease

Continuous education on Wilson disease is vital for both patients and caregivers to manage the condition effectively. Staying informed about the latest research, treatment options, and lifestyle adjustments can empower patients to take an active role in their care. Resources such as online courses, webinars, and workshops can provide valuable information and support.

Patients should regularly consult reliable sources, including medical professionals and reputable organizations, to stay updated on their condition. Engaging with the latest developments can enhance understanding and improve health outcomes, allowing individuals to make informed decisions regarding their treatment and lifestyle.

Resources for Emergency Contacts and Support

Having a comprehensive list of emergency contacts and support resources is essential for individuals with Wilson disease. This list should include healthcare providers, local emergency services, and national helplines. Patients and caregivers should ensure this information is easily accessible in case of emergencies.

In addition to emergency contacts, patients can benefit from support resources such as local support groups or online forums dedicated to Wilson disease. These communities offer a platform for sharing experiences, seeking advice, and finding emotional support, helping individuals feel less isolated in their journey.

Discussion on Palliative Care Options

Palliative care options can play an important role in improving the quality of life for individuals with Wilson disease experiencing significant symptoms or complications. This approach focuses on providing relief from symptoms and stress rather than attempting to cure the disease. Patients should discuss their preferences for palliative care with their healthcare team to ensure they receive comprehensive support.

To access palliative care services, patients can consult their primary healthcare provider or seek referrals from specialists. Integrating palliative care into the treatment plan can enhance symptom management and emotional support, ultimately improving overall well-being.

Success Stories of Patients Overcoming Complications

Learning from success stories of patients who have overcome complications related to Wilson disease can provide hope and inspiration. Many individuals share their journeys of navigating challenges, utilizing effective management strategies, and advocating for their health. These stories often highlight the importance of a strong support system, adherence to treatment plans, and open communication with healthcare providers.

Patients can find these success stories through online forums, support groups, or advocacy organizations. Engaging with these narratives can empower others facing similar challenges, demonstrating that with proper management and support, it is possible to live a fulfilling life while managing Wilson disease.

CHAPTER 9:

Living with Wilson Disease

Importance of Acceptance and Adaptation

Accepting Wilson disease is a vital first step in managing the disorder effectively. Acceptance involves understanding the condition, its implications, and how it may affect daily life. This emotional adjustment can reduce anxiety and improve mental well-being, allowing individuals to focus on managing their health rather than feeling overwhelmed by their diagnosis. Adapting involves making necessary lifestyle changes, including medication adherence and dietary adjustments, which can help in effectively managing the disease and minimizing symptoms.

To adapt successfully, individuals can establish a routine that incorporates treatment regimens, exercise, and healthy eating. Building a support system—whether through family, friends, or support groups—can further aid in the adaptation process. Practical tools such as journals can help track symptoms and progress, reinforcing positive changes and highlighting areas for further improvement.

Strategies for Maintaining a Positive Outlook

Maintaining a positive outlook is essential for managing Wilson disease. Practicing mindfulness and gratitude can shift focus from negative aspects of the condition to the positives in life. Engaging in activities that bring joy, such as hobbies, socializing, or volunteering, can foster a sense of purpose and happiness. Regularly reminding oneself of personal strengths and past accomplishments can also help build resilience in the face of challenges.

Additionally, setting realistic goals can provide motivation and a sense of achievement. This could include small daily tasks or larger long-term aspirations. Embracing a problem-solving mindset, where challenges are viewed as opportunities for growth, can significantly contribute to a more positive perspective on living with Wilson disease.

Importance of Celebrating Small Victories

Celebrating small victories is crucial in maintaining motivation and morale when managing Wilson disease. Recognizing and acknowledging progress, no matter how minor, can help reinforce positive behaviors and attitudes. This could be as simple as successfully following a dietary guideline for a week or achieving a minor health milestone, like improved lab results. Each victory serves as a reminder of one's ability to manage the condition effectively.

To implement this, individuals can keep a victory log where they document achievements and positive experiences. Sharing these victories with supportive friends or family can further amplify the sense of accomplishment and foster a communal environment of encouragement and celebration.

Overview of Long-Term Prognosis with Treatment

With appropriate treatment and lifestyle management, individuals with Wilson disease can lead healthy and fulfilling lives. Early diagnosis and adherence to prescribed therapies, including chelating agents and zinc supplements, are crucial in preventing copper accumulation and mitigating potential organ damage. Regular monitoring by healthcare professionals ensures timely adjustments to treatment plans, which can improve long-term health outcomes.

Long-term prognosis varies among individuals, but many report improved symptoms and overall health with consistent treatment. Staying informed about the disease and actively participating in one's healthcare decisions can empower individuals to take control of their health and maintain a positive outlook regarding their prognosis.

Importance of Community Involvement and Activism

Community involvement plays a pivotal role in raising awareness about Wilson disease and promoting better resources and support for affected individuals. Engaging in local or national advocacy groups can help individuals connect with others facing similar challenges and contribute to initiatives aimed at improving care and research funding. This involvement can enhance a sense of belonging and purpose while amplifying the voices of those impacted by the disease.

Taking part in community events, fundraising activities, or awareness campaigns can create a powerful platform for education and advocacy. By sharing personal experiences, individuals can contribute to a broader understanding of Wilson disease, fostering empathy and support within their communities while also driving impactful change.

Encouragement for Sharing Experiences with Others

Sharing experiences with others can be incredibly beneficial for individuals living with Wilson disease. Opening up about personal journeys fosters connection and provides emotional relief, as it can help diminish feelings of isolation. Online forums, support groups, or even casual conversations with friends and family can offer a safe space for discussing challenges, successes, and coping strategies.

Encouragement to share should also extend to platforms where individuals can write about their experiences, whether through blogs, social media, or community newsletters. This not only helps others who may feel alone but can also empower the storyteller, reinforcing their resilience and ability to manage the disorder.

Strategies for Finding Joy in Daily Life

Finding joy in daily life is essential for maintaining a positive mental state while managing Wilson disease. This can involve creating daily rituals that incorporate activities that bring happiness, such as engaging in favorite hobbies, spending time with loved ones, or practicing mindfulness techniques. It's important to make time for self-care, which can include physical activities, creative pursuits, or relaxation exercises, all of which contribute to overall well-being.

Additionally, setting small, enjoyable goals each day can provide motivation and a sense of accomplishment. Whether it's trying a new recipe that aligns with dietary restrictions or planning a short outing, focusing on joyful experiences can enhance quality of life and serve as a reminder of what brings happiness amidst the challenges of living with the condition.

Importance of Continuing Education on Wilson Disease

Continuing education about Wilson disease is vital for effective self-management and staying informed about the latest research and treatment options. Individuals can utilize reputable resources, such as medical websites, peer-reviewed journals, and patient organizations, to deepen their understanding of the condition. Engaging in educational seminars, webinars, or workshops can also provide valuable insights into managing symptoms and improving health outcomes.

By remaining proactive in education, individuals can advocate for their health and make informed decisions regarding their treatment and care. Knowledge empowers individuals to navigate their journey with Wilson disease more effectively and enhances their ability to communicate with healthcare providers about their needs and concerns.

Patient Stories of Hope and Perseverance

Hearing patient stories of hope and perseverance can be incredibly motivating for those diagnosed with Wilson disease. These narratives often highlight the resilience and determination of individuals who have successfully managed their condition despite challenges. Sharing stories can foster a sense of community and provide practical strategies and inspiration for navigating similar struggles.

Patients can seek out these inspiring stories through blogs, podcasts, or support groups. Connecting with others who have overcome obstacles can instill a sense of hope and encourage individuals to remain committed to their treatment plans and embrace their journey with positivity and strength.

Importance of Planning for the Future

Planning for the future is crucial for individuals living with Wilson disease, as it allows them to set personal and health-related goals. This can include making decisions about career aspirations, family planning, and long-term health management strategies. Having a plan in place can provide a sense of control and direction, which is essential for mental well-being.

Involving healthcare professionals in this planning process can enhance understanding of how Wilson disease may impact future choices. Creating contingency plans for potential health changes can also prepare individuals for various scenarios, ensuring they have resources and support readily available as they navigate their journey.

Resources for Lifelong Learning about Wilson Disease

Utilizing resources for lifelong learning about Wilson disease is essential for effective self-management. Various organizations provide comprehensive information about the condition, including educational materials, support networks, and updates on research advancements. Online platforms, support groups, and patient advocacy organizations can be valuable resources for individuals seeking knowledge and community.

Regularly accessing credible sources ensures that individuals stay informed about the latest treatment options, dietary recommendations, and management strategies. This continuous learning process can empower patients to advocate for their health, make informed decisions, and feel more confident in navigating the complexities of living with Wilson disease.

Encouragement for Family Involvement in Care

Family involvement in care is crucial for individuals with Wilson disease, as it provides emotional support and practical assistance in managing the condition. Educating family members about the disease can foster understanding and empathy, allowing them to participate meaningfully in care routines and decision-making processes. This support network can enhance adherence to treatment plans and create a collaborative environment for managing health.

Encouraging open communication among family members about challenges and needs can strengthen these support systems. Regular family meetings or discussions can help address concerns, celebrate successes, and reinforce the commitment to managing Wilson disease together, fostering a sense of unity and shared purpose.

Final Thoughts on Living Fully with Wilson Disease

Living fully with Wilson disease involves embracing life while effectively managing the condition. This requires a proactive approach to treatment, self-care, and mental well-being. Building a strong support network, setting realistic goals, and continuously educating oneself can significantly enhance quality of life. Individuals are encouraged to focus on personal passions and cultivate joy in everyday experiences, allowing them to thrive despite the challenges posed by the disorder.

By adopting a holistic approach that prioritizes health, happiness, and community involvement, individuals with Wilson disease can lead fulfilling lives. Embracing the journey, sharing experiences, and celebrating victories—both big and small—further enrich the experience of living with this condition, creating a meaningful and empowered life.

Common Concerns

Can Wilson Disease be cured?

Wilson Disease currently has no known cure, but it is manageable with proper treatment and lifestyle adjustments. Treatment typically involves medications that help remove excess copper from the body, such as chelating agents (e.g., penicillamine) and zinc, which can reduce copper absorption. Regular monitoring by a healthcare provider is crucial to adjust treatment as needed and to prevent complications associated with copper buildup.

Although a cure isn't available, early detection and consistent management can lead to a normal life expectancy and a reduction in symptoms. Individuals must commit to lifelong treatment and regular follow-ups with their healthcare team to manage the disease effectively and minimize organ damage.

What lifestyle changes are essential for managing symptoms?

Managing Wilson Disease requires significant lifestyle changes to reduce copper intake and promote liver health. It is essential to avoid copper-rich foods, such as shellfish, nuts, chocolate, and organ meats. Instead, focus on a balanced diet rich in fruits, vegetables, and whole grains while ensuring adequate hydration. Consulting with a registered dietitian can help create a tailored meal plan that supports copper management.

In addition to dietary adjustments, maintaining regular medical appointments for blood tests and liver function monitoring is vital. Engaging in regular physical activity and managing stress through techniques like yoga or meditation can also enhance overall well-being and help mitigate some symptoms associated with Wilson Disease.

How does Wilson Disease affect daily life and relationships?

Wilson Disease can significantly impact daily life, as individuals may experience various physical and emotional symptoms, such as fatigue, cognitive difficulties, or mood swings. These symptoms can interfere with work, social activities, and personal relationships. Open communication with family and friends about the condition can foster understanding and support, making it easier to navigate challenges together.

To cope with these impacts, individuals should consider establishing a routine that includes time for self-care, hobbies, and social interactions. This structure can provide a sense of normalcy and help manage stress levels, ultimately improving relationships and overall quality of life.

Are there support groups for individuals with Wilson Disease?

Yes, numerous support groups and organizations are dedicated to helping individuals with Wilson Disease and their families. These groups provide valuable resources, information, and emotional support through shared experiences. Connecting with others facing similar challenges can alleviate feelings of isolation and provide practical coping strategies.

Online forums, local chapters, and national organizations, such as the Wilson Disease Association, offer opportunities for individuals to engage in discussions, share experiences, and access educational materials. Participating in these communities can be instrumental in managing the condition and fostering connections with others who understand the journey.

What should I do if I experience new symptoms?

If you experience new or worsening symptoms related to Wilson Disease, it is crucial to contact your healthcare provider immediately. Keeping a detailed journal of your symptoms, including their onset, duration, and any triggers, can help your doctor assess your situation more effectively. Promptly addressing new symptoms can prevent further complications and allow for timely adjustments in your treatment plan.

In addition to contacting your healthcare provider, consider reaching out to your support network for emotional assistance. Sharing your concerns with family and friends can provide comfort and help you feel less overwhelmed. Remember, proactive communication with your healthcare team is vital for effective management of Wilson Disease.

What is Wilson Disease?

Wilson Disease is a rare genetic disorder that leads to the abnormal accumulation of copper in the body, particularly in the liver, brain, and other vital organs. This buildup can result from a defect in the ATP7B gene, which is responsible for copper transport and excretion. As copper levels rise, they can cause serious health issues, including liver disease, neurological disorders, and psychiatric symptoms.

Individuals diagnosed with Wilson Disease typically experience a range of symptoms, including fatigue, jaundice, abdominal pain, and movement disorders. Understanding the nature of this disorder is essential for effective management and treatment, as early intervention can significantly improve outcomes.

How is Wilson Disease diagnosed?

The diagnosis of Wilson Disease involves a combination of clinical evaluations, medical history, and laboratory tests. Blood tests can measure serum copper levels, ceruloplasmin levels, and liver function indicators. Additionally, 24-hour urine tests can assess copper excretion, providing insights into copper overload in the body.

In some cases, a liver biopsy may be required to measure copper concentration directly from liver tissue. This procedure, while invasive, can provide definitive evidence of copper accumulation and help healthcare providers determine the most effective treatment approach.

What are the common symptoms of Wilson Disease?

Common symptoms of Wilson Disease can vary widely, often appearing in late childhood or early adulthood. Physical symptoms may include abdominal pain, jaundice, swelling, and liver dysfunction. Neurological symptoms can manifest as tremors, difficulty speaking or swallowing, and changes in personality or behavior, making it challenging to recognize the disorder without proper testing.

Psychiatric symptoms, such as anxiety, depression, or mood swings, may also occur, complicating the clinical picture. Understanding these symptoms is crucial for early detection and intervention, allowing individuals to seek appropriate care and implement necessary lifestyle changes for effective management.

Conclusion

Wilson Disease is a manageable condition with the right knowledge, treatment, and support. Early diagnosis and proactive lifestyle adjustments can significantly improve quality of life and prevent severe complications. By understanding the disease, making informed choices, and fostering a supportive environment, individuals with Wilson Disease can lead fulfilling lives.